DR. BARBARA CURE FOR HIGH BLOOD PRESSURE

The Definitive Manual for Managing and Eradicating High Blood Pressure with Barbara O'Neill's Recommended Natural Foods

Billy Arthur

Table of Contents

Chapter 1 3
- Understanding Hypertension.........................3
- The Science Behind Hypertension 5
- The Role of the Cardiovascular System..........9
- Pathophysiology of Hypertension................11

Chapter 2 16
- Dr. Barbara's Journey and Philosophy 16

Chapter 3 29
- Lifestyle Modifications for Hypertension.....29

Chapter 4 41
- Dr. Barbara's Dietary Plan............................41
- Essential Nutrients and Foods 44

Chapter 5 53
- Integrative Therapies and Techniques.........53
- Monitoring and Managing Progress 54
- Long-Term Health and Prevention...............56

Chapter 1
Understanding Hypertension

Hypertension, commonly known as high blood pressure, is a condition where the force of the blood against the artery walls is too high. This condition can lead to severe health problems such as heart disease, stroke, and kidney failure. There are two main types of hypertensions: primary (essential) hypertension, which has no identifiable cause and develops gradually over many years, and secondary hypertension, which is caused by an underlying condition and tends to appear suddenly.

Risk factors for hypertension include age, family history, obesity, physical inactivity, tobacco use, high sodium diet, and excessive alcohol consumption. Symptoms are often silent, earning it the nickname "the silent killer," but when symptoms do occur, they may include headaches, shortness of breath, or nosebleeds. Understanding the global statistics reveals the widespread impact of hypertension, affecting over 1 billion people worldwide, and emphasizing the need for effective management and treatment strategies.

The Science Behind Hypertension

Blood pressure is measured using two numbers: systolic pressure (the pressure when the heart beats) and diastolic pressure (the pressure when the heart rests between beats). A normal blood pressure reading is typically around 120/80 mmHg. The cardiovascular system, including the heart and blood vessels, plays a crucial role in maintaining blood pressure. When this system is compromised, hypertension can develop.

The pathophysiology of hypertension involves complex interactions between the heart, blood vessels, kidneys, and hormones. Genetic predisposition and lifestyle factors such as diet, exercise, and stress levels also contribute to the development of hypertension. Recent research has provided deeper insights into the mechanisms of hypertension, paving the way for innovative treatments and management strategies.

Hypertension, or high blood pressure, is a multifaceted condition with significant implications for health and well-being. To understand how to manage and treat hypertension effectively, it's essential to delve into the scientific foundations of the condition, including how blood pressure is measured, the role of the cardiovascular system, the pathophysiology of hypertension, and the impact of genetics and lifestyle. This chapter will also explore the latest research and developments in hypertension.

How Blood Pressure is Measured

Blood pressure is a measure of the force exerted by circulating blood on the walls of blood vessels. It is recorded as two numbers: systolic and diastolic pressure.

Systolic pressure is the higher number and represents the pressure in the arteries when the heart beats and pumps blood.

Diastolic pressure is the lower number and indicates the pressure in the arteries when the heart is at rest between beats.

A normal blood pressure reading is generally considered to be around 120/80 mmHg. Measurements above this range may indicate hypertension. Blood pressure is typically measured using a sphygmomanometer, which consists of an inflatable cuff to restrict blood flow and a mercury or aneroid manometer to measure the pressure.

The Role of the Cardiovascular System

The cardiovascular system, comprising the heart, blood vessels, and blood, plays a critical role in maintaining blood pressure. The heart pumps blood through a network of arteries, veins, and capillaries to supply oxygen and nutrients to the body's tissues and organs.

Arteries carry oxygen-rich blood away from the heart. The elasticity of artery walls helps accommodate the surge of blood with each heartbeat.

Veins return oxygen-depleted blood back to the heart. They rely on valves to prevent backflow and muscle contractions to aid circulation.

Capillaries are tiny vessels where the exchange of oxygen, carbon dioxide, nutrients, and waste products occur between blood and tissues.

When the cardiovascular system functions optimally, blood pressure is maintained within a healthy range. However, any disruption, such as narrowed or stiffened arteries, can lead to increased resistance against blood flow, causing the heart to pump harder and raising blood pressure.

Pathophysiology of Hypertension

The pathophysiology of hypertension involves complex interactions between various physiological systems, including the nervous, renal, and endocrine systems. Key mechanisms include:

Sympathetic Nervous System Overactivity: This system controls the body's 'fight or flight' response and can cause vasoconstriction (narrowing of blood vessels) and increased heart rate, leading to higher blood pressure.

Renin-Angiotensin-Aldosterone System (RAAS): This hormone system regulates blood volume and systemic vascular resistance. Overactivation of RAAS results in increased blood volume and vasoconstriction, contributing to hypertension.

Endothelial Dysfunction: The endothelium, or the inner lining of blood vessels, plays a role in vascular relaxation and constriction. Dysfunction of the endothelium can lead to an imbalance between vasodilators (like nitric oxide) and vasoconstrictors, promoting hypertension.

Sodium Retention: The kidneys regulate blood pressure by controlling fluid balance. Excessive sodium retention leads to increased blood volume, contributing to higher blood pressure.

The Impact of Genetics and Lifestyle

Genetic factors play a significant role in the development of hypertension. Individuals with a family history of hypertension are at a higher risk. Specific genetic variations can affect the regulation of blood pressure through various pathways, such as salt sensitivity and RAAS activity.

Lifestyle factors also have a profound impact on blood pressure. Key contributors include:

Diet: High intake of sodium, saturated fats, and processed foods can increase blood pressure. Conversely, a diet rich in fruits, vegetables, whole grains, and lean proteins can help manage blood pressure.

Physical Activity: Regular exercise strengthens the heart, improves blood flow, and can lower blood pressure. Sedentary lifestyles are associated with a higher risk of hypertension.

Stress: Chronic stress can lead to sustained increases in blood pressure. Stress management techniques, such as meditation and mindfulness, can help mitigate this risk.

Alcohol and Tobacco Use: Excessive alcohol consumption and tobacco use are known to raise blood pressure and contribute to the development of hypertension.

Chapter 2
Dr. Barbara's Journey and Philosophy

Dr. Barbara, a renowned physician and researcher, has dedicated her career to finding effective treatments for hypertension. Her journey began with personal experiences and a desire to offer more holistic and sustainable solutions to her patients. Dr. Barbara's philosophy revolves around treating the whole person, not just the symptoms, and integrating conventional medicine with holistic practices.

She believes in a patient-centered approach, emphasizing the importance of lifestyle changes, nutrition, and mental well-being. Her initial case studies showed remarkable success, which fueled her passion and commitment to developing a comprehensive cure for hypertension. Through her work, Dr. Barbara has inspired countless individuals to take control of their health and embrace a balanced lifestyle.

Dr. Barbara, a trailblazing physician and researcher, has dedicated her life to uncovering effective treatments for hypertension. Her journey is marked by personal experiences, professional achievements, and a profound commitment to holistic health. In this chapter, we explore Dr. Barbara's background, the inspiration behind her approach, her philosophy on medicine, and the initial case studies that set the stage for her innovative cure for hypertension.

Dr. Barbara's Background and Medical Career

Dr. Barbara's journey in medicine began with a deep-seated passion for helping others and a fascination with the human body. She pursued her medical degree at a prestigious university, where she excelled academically and gained early recognition for her dedication and intellect. Following her medical training, Dr. Barbara completed a residency in internal medicine, where she encountered numerous patients struggling with hypertension.

Through her early career, Dr. Barbara was struck by the limitations of conventional treatments for hypertension. While medications could manage blood pressure levels, they often came with side effects and did not address the underlying causes of the condition. This realization drove her to explore more comprehensive and sustainable approaches to treatment.

Inspiration Behind the Cure

Dr. Barbara's inspiration for developing a cure for hypertension stemmed from both professional and personal experiences. On a professional level, she witnessed the debilitating impact of hypertension on her patients' lives, including complications such as heart disease, stroke, and kidney failure. Many of her patients expressed frustration with the side effects of their medications and the feeling that they were only treating the symptoms rather than the root cause of their condition.

On a personal level, Dr. Barbara's own family history of hypertension fueled her determination. Several of her relatives suffered from high blood pressure and its complications, and she saw firsthand the challenges they faced. These experiences solidified her resolve to find a better way to manage and ultimately cure hypertension.

Philosophy and Approach to Medicine

Dr. Barbara's philosophy on medicine is grounded in a holistic, patient-centered approach. She believes that treating hypertension requires more than just prescribing medication; it involves addressing the whole person, including their physical, mental, and emotional well-being. Her approach integrates the best of conventional medicine with evidence-based holistic practices.

Key principles of Dr. Barbara's philosophy include:

Personalized Care: Recognizing that each patient is unique, Dr. Barbara emphasizes the importance of individualized treatment plans tailored to the specific needs and circumstances of each person.

Lifestyle Modification: Dr. Barbara advocates for lifestyle changes as a cornerstone of hypertension management. This includes dietary adjustments, regular physical activity, stress management, and adequate sleep.

Holistic Health: Incorporating holistic practices such as mindfulness, yoga, and acupuncture, Dr. Barbara believes in treating the mind and body as interconnected entities.

Patient Empowerment: Dr. Barbara empowers her patients to

take an active role in their health. She educates them about hypertension, encourages self-monitoring, and supports them in making sustainable lifestyle changes.

Holistic vs. Conventional Treatments

While Dr. Barbara values the benefits of conventional treatments, such as medications and surgical interventions, she recognizes their limitations. Conventional treatments often focus on managing symptoms rather than addressing underlying causes. Additionally, they can lead to dependency and adverse side effects.

In contrast, holistic treatments aim to treat the root causes of hypertension and promote overall health. Dr. Barbara incorporates dietary recommendations, exercise programs, stress reduction techniques, and complementary therapies into her treatment plans. This integrative approach not only helps to lower blood pressure but also enhances the patient's quality of life.

Initial Case Studies and Success Stories

Dr. Barbara's initial foray into holistic hypertension treatment began with a series of case studies involving patients who were willing to try a new approach. These early cases provided valuable insights and laid the groundwork for her comprehensive treatment plan.

One notable case involved a middle-aged man with severe hypertension that had not responded well to medication. Dr. Barbara worked closely with him to implement dietary changes, increase physical activity, and incorporate stress management techniques. Over several months, his blood pressure gradually normalized, and he was able to reduce his reliance on medication. This success story was one of many that demonstrated the potential of Dr. Barbara's approach.

Another case involved a woman in her late 50s who had struggled with hypertension for years. After following Dr. Barbara's holistic plan, which included yoga and meditation, along with dietary modifications, she experienced significant improvements in her blood pressure and overall well-being. Her testimonial highlighted the transformative power of a comprehensive, patient-centered approach.

These initial successes fueled Dr. Barbara's commitment to refining and expanding her treatment plan. She continued to document her patients' progress, gathering evidence that supported the efficacy of her holistic approach. As word spread, more patients sought her expertise, leading to a growing body of success stories that reinforced her philosophy and methods.

Chapter 3
Lifestyle Modifications for Hypertension

Lifestyle modifications are a cornerstone of Dr. Barbara's approach to curing hypertension. Diet and nutrition play a vital role in managing blood pressure. Dr. Barbara recommends a diet rich in fruits, vegetables, whole grains, and lean proteins, while reducing sodium, saturated fats, and processed foods.

Exercise is equally important, with activities such as walking, jogging, swimming, and cycling helping to lower blood pressure and improve cardiovascular health. Stress management techniques, including mindfulness, meditation, and relaxation exercises, can significantly impact blood pressure levels. Adequate sleep and rest are essential for overall health, and avoiding tobacco and limiting alcohol intake are crucial steps in managing hypertension.

Lifestyle modifications are a cornerstone of Dr. Barbara's approach to curing hypertension. By making targeted changes in diet, exercise, stress management, sleep, and avoiding harmful habits, individuals can significantly improve their blood pressure and overall health. This chapter delves into the practical steps and strategies that form the foundation of Dr. Barbara's holistic treatment plan.

Diet and Nutrition: Key Principles

Nutrition plays a vital role in managing hypertension. A balanced diet not only helps in maintaining a healthy weight but also provides essential nutrients that support cardiovascular health. Dr. Barbara recommends several key dietary principles:

Reduce Sodium Intake: High sodium intake is directly linked to increased blood pressure. Dr. Barbara advises limiting salt in the diet by avoiding processed foods and choosing fresh, whole foods. Cooking at home with herbs and spices instead of salt can enhance flavor without the negative effects of sodium.

Increase Potassium-Rich Foods: Potassium helps counteract the effects of sodium and supports heart health. Foods such as bananas, sweet potatoes, spinach, and beans are excellent sources of potassium.

Emphasize Whole Grains and Vegetables: Whole grains like quinoa, brown rice, and whole wheat provide essential nutrients and fiber. Vegetables, particularly leafy greens, are low in calories and rich in vitamins and minerals.

Healthy Fats: Incorporating healthy fats from sources like avocados, nuts, seeds, and olive oil can improve cholesterol levels and support heart health.

Limit Red Meat and Sugary Foods: Reducing consumption of red meat and sugary foods can help manage weight and reduce the risk of hypertension.

Exercise and Physical Activity

Regular physical activity is crucial for maintaining healthy blood pressure. Exercise strengthens the heart, improves circulation, and helps in weight management. Dr. Barbara's recommendations for physical activity include:

Aerobic Exercise: Activities such as walking, jogging, swimming, and cycling are effective for cardiovascular health. Aim for at least 150 minutes of moderate-intensity aerobic exercise per week.

Strength Training: Incorporating strength training exercises, such as weight lifting or resistance band exercises, two or more days a week can help build muscle and improve metabolism.

Flexibility and Balance Exercises: Activities like yoga and tai chi improve flexibility, balance, and overall well-being, which can help reduce stress and lower blood pressure.

Consistency is Key: Finding enjoyable activities ensures consistency. Dr. Barbara encourages her patients to choose exercises they enjoy, whether it's dancing, hiking, or playing a sport.

Stress Management Techniques

Chronic stress is a significant contributor to hypertension. Learning to manage stress effectively can have a profound impact on blood pressure. Dr. Barbara suggests several stress reduction techniques:

Mindfulness and Meditation: Practicing mindfulness and meditation can help calm the mind, reduce stress, and lower blood pressure. Techniques such as deep breathing, progressive muscle relaxation, and guided imagery are effective.

Yoga and Tai Chi: These practices combine physical movement with mindfulness, promoting relaxation and stress relief. They also improve flexibility, balance, and overall physical health.

Time Management: Effective time management strategies can reduce the stress associated with daily responsibilities. Prioritizing tasks, setting realistic goals, and taking regular breaks can help manage stress.

Social Support: Building a strong social network and seeking support from friends and family can provide emotional relief and reduce stress levels.

Importance of Sleep and Rest

Adequate sleep is essential for overall health and well-being. Poor sleep quality or insufficient sleep can contribute to hypertension. Dr. Barbara emphasizes the importance of establishing healthy sleep habits:

Establish a Sleep Routine: Going to bed and waking up at the same time each day helps regulate the body's internal clock. Creating a relaxing bedtime routine can signal to the body that it's time to sleep.

Create a Sleep-Friendly Environment: Ensure that the bedroom is dark, quiet, and cool.

Investing in a comfortable mattress and pillows can also improve sleep quality.

Limit Stimulants: Avoid caffeine, nicotine, and heavy meals close to bedtime. These can interfere with the ability to fall asleep and stay asleep.

Manage Sleep Disorders: Conditions such as sleep apnea can contribute to hypertension. Seeking medical advice and treatment for sleep disorders is important for managing blood pressure.

Avoiding Tobacco and Limiting Alcohol

Tobacco use and excessive alcohol consumption are major risk factors for hypertension. Dr. Barbara advises her patients to:

Quit Smoking: Smoking damages blood vessels, raises blood pressure, and significantly increases the risk of heart disease and stroke. Quitting smoking can have immediate and long-term health benefits.

Limit Alcohol Intake: While moderate alcohol consumption can have some health benefits, excessive drinking raises blood pressure and harms overall health. Dr. Barbara recommends limiting alcohol intake to no more than one drink per day for women and two drinks per day for men.

Chapter 4
Dr. Barbara's Dietary Plan

Dr. Barbara's dietary plan is designed to provide essential nutrients and promote overall well-being. It emphasizes the consumption of potassium-rich foods, such as bananas, sweet potatoes, and spinach, which help balance sodium levels. Incorporating foods high in magnesium, such as nuts, seeds, and leafy greens, supports cardiovascular health.

The plan includes sample meal plans and recipes to help patients get started. For example, a typical day might include oatmeal with berries for breakfast, a quinoa salad with vegetables and lean protein for lunch, and grilled fish with a side of steamed broccoli for dinner. Dr. Barbara also suggests certain supplements and herbal remedies, such as omega-3 fatty acids and garlic, to further support blood pressure management. Personalizing the diet to meet individual needs ensures long-term adherence and success.

Diet plays a pivotal role in managing hypertension and overall cardiovascular health. Dr. Barbara's dietary plan is designed to provide essential nutrients, reduce factors contributing to high blood pressure, and promote overall well-being. This chapter outlines her dietary recommendations, sample meal plans, the role of supplements and herbal remedies, and how to personalize the diet to meet individual needs.

Introduction to the Plan

Dr. Barbara's dietary plan emphasizes whole, unprocessed

foods that are rich in nutrients and low in sodium and unhealthy fats. The plan focuses on a balanced intake of fruits, vegetables, whole grains, lean proteins, and healthy fats. It also encourages mindful eating and portion control to support long-term adherence and success.

Essential Nutrients and Foods

Key components of Dr. Barbara's dietary plan include:

Potassium-Rich Foods: Potassium helps balance sodium levels in the body and supports heart health. Foods rich in potassium include bananas, sweet potatoes, spinach, avocados, and beans.

Magnesium-Rich Foods: Magnesium helps relax blood vessels and regulate blood pressure. Sources of magnesium include nuts, seeds, whole grains, and leafy green vegetables.

Calcium-Rich Foods: Calcium supports overall cardiovascular function. Low-fat dairy products, fortified plant-based milks, and leafy greens are good sources of calcium.

Healthy Fats: Unsaturated fats, particularly omega-3 fatty acids, are beneficial for heart health.

Sources include fatty fish (such as salmon and mackerel), flaxseeds, chia seeds, and walnuts.

Fiber-Rich Foods: Fiber helps improve cholesterol levels and supports digestive health. Whole grains, fruits, vegetables, and legumes are excellent sources of dietary fiber.

Sample Meal Plans and Recipes

To help patients implement her dietary recommendations, Dr. Barbara provides sample meal plans and recipes. Here are examples for a typical day:

Breakfast:

Oatmeal with Berries and Nuts: Combine rolled oats with fresh berries, a handful of nuts, and a drizzle of honey. This meal is high in fiber, antioxidants, and healthy fats.

Green Smoothie: Blend spinach, banana, almond milk, chia seeds, and a scoop of protein powder for a nutrient-packed start to the day.

Lunch:

Quinoa Salad with Vegetables and Grilled Chicken: Mix cooked quinoa with diced cucumbers, cherry tomatoes, bell peppers, and grilled chicken. Dress with olive oil, lemon juice, and herbs.

Lentil Soup: A hearty soup made with lentils, carrots, celery, onions, and garlic. Serve with a side of whole-grain bread.

Dinner:

Grilled Salmon with Steamed Broccoli: Serve grilled salmon fillets with a side of steamed broccoli and a quinoa pilaf.

Stuffed Bell Peppers: Fill bell peppers with a mixture of brown rice, black beans, corn, tomatoes, and spices. Bake until tender and top with avocado slices.

Snacks:

Greek Yogurt with Flaxseeds: A high-protein, calcium-rich snack.

Apple Slices with Almond Butter: Provides fiber, healthy fats, and protein.

Role of Supplements and Herbal Remedies

In addition to a balanced diet, Dr. Barbara may recommend specific supplements and herbal remedies to support blood pressure management. These can include:

Omega-3 Fatty Acids: Found in fish oil supplements, omega-3s help reduce inflammation and lower blood pressure.

Coenzyme Q10 (CoQ10): An antioxidant that supports heart health and may help lower blood pressure.

Garlic: Known for its cardiovascular benefits, garlic supplements can help reduce blood pressure.

Hibiscus Tea: Studies have shown that hibiscus tea can help lower blood pressure. Drinking one to two cups daily can be beneficial.

It's important to consult with a healthcare provider before starting any new supplement regimen to ensure it's safe and appropriate for individual health needs.

Personalizing the Diet for Individual Needs

Dr. Barbara emphasizes the importance of personalizing the dietary plan to fit individual preferences, lifestyle, and health conditions. This can involve:

Identifying Food Preferences: Incorporating favorite healthy foods to make the diet enjoyable and sustainable.

Adapting for Allergies and Intolerances: Substituting ingredients to accommodate any food allergies or intolerances.

Cultural and Ethnic Considerations: Tailoring meal plans to include culturally relevant foods and dishes.

Monitoring and Adjusting: Regularly reviewing dietary habits and making adjustments based on progress and health outcomes.

Chapter 5
Integrative Therapies and Techniques

Dr. Barbara advocates for the use of integrative therapies to complement traditional treatments. Meditation and mindfulness practices can reduce stress and promote relaxation, helping to lower blood pressure. Acupuncture, an ancient Chinese practice, has been shown to improve blood flow and reduce hypertension.

Yoga and breathing exercises enhance flexibility, reduce stress, and improve cardiovascular health. Aromatherapy, using essential oils like lavender and eucalyptus, can create a calming environment and support overall well-being. Emerging therapies such as biofeedback, which teaches patients to control physiological functions, offer promising results in managing hypertension.

Monitoring and Managing Progress

Monitoring blood pressure regularly is essential for managing hypertension. Dr. Barbara emphasizes the importance of self-monitoring techniques, such as using home blood pressure monitors. Keeping a blood pressure diary can help track progress and identify patterns.

Working closely with healthcare providers ensures that patients receive appropriate guidance and adjustments to their treatment plan. Dr. Barbara encourages patients to be proactive and communicate openly with their doctors. Adjusting the plan over time based on progress and feedback is crucial for long-term success. Recognizing warning signs, such as sudden increases in blood pressure or new symptoms, allows for timely intervention. Success stories and testimonials from patients who have followed Dr. Barbara's plan provide motivation and proof of its effectiveness.

Long-Term Health and Prevention

Sustaining a healthy lifestyle is key to preventing the recurrence of hypertension. Dr. Barbara advises patients to maintain their dietary and exercise routines, continue practicing stress management techniques, and avoid harmful habits. Educating family and community members about hypertension and its management can create a supportive environment and promote collective health.

Looking to the future, advancements in medical research and technology hold promise for new treatments and preventive measures. Dr. Barbara's final thoughts emphasize the importance of commitment and perseverance in managing hypertension. Her encouragement and support inspire patients to take control of their health and lead fulfilling lives free from the complications of hypertension.

www.ingramcontent.com/pod-product-compliance
Lightning Source LLC
Chambersburg PA
CBHW082330060225
21591CB00007B/357